My Exercise Log

Name   _____

Telephone No.   _____

Email   _____

Address   _____

                  _____

Name of Doctor   _____

Doctor's No.   _____

My Goals

Goal Weight: _____

Goal Period _____

Notes

_____

_____

_____

_____

_____

_____

_____

_____

_____

_____

_____

_____

Exercise Log

Date	Weight	Exercise/ Activity	Time	Notes

Exercise Log

Date	Weight	Exercise/ Activity	Time	Notes

Exercise Log

Date	Weight	Exercise/ Activity	Time	Notes

Exercise Log

Date	Weight	Exercise/ Activity	Time	Notes

Exercise Log

Date	Weight	Exercise/ Activity	Time	Notes

Exercise Log

Date	Weight	Exercise/ Activity	Time	Notes

Exercise Log

Date	Weight	Exercise/ Activity	Time	Notes

Exercise Log

Date	Weight	Exercise/ Activity	Time	Notes

Exercise Log

Date	Weight	Exercise/ Activity	Time	Notes

Exercise Log

Date	Weight	Exercise/ Activity	Time	Notes

Exercise Log

Date	Weight	Exercise/ Activity	Time	Notes

Exercise Log

Date	Weight	Exercise/ Activity	Time	Notes

Exercise Log

Date	Weight	Exercise/ Activity	Time	Notes

Exercise Log

Date	Weight	Exercise/ Activity	Time	Notes

Exercise Log

Date	Weight	Exercise/ Activity	Time	Notes

Exercise Log

Date	Weight	Exercise/ Activity	Time	Notes

Exercise Log

Date	Weight	Exercise/ Activity	Time	Notes

Exercise Log

Date	Weight	Exercise/ Activity	Time	Notes

Exercise Log

Date	Weight	Exercise/ Activity	Time	Notes

Exercise Log

Date	Weight	Exercise/ Activity	Time	Notes

Exercise Log

Date	Weight	Exercise/ Activity	Time	Notes

Exercise Log

Date	Weight	Exercise/ Activity	Time	Notes

Exercise Log

Date	Weight	Exercise/ Activity	Time	Notes

Exercise Log

Date	Weight	Exercise/ Activity	Time	Notes

Exercise Log

Date	Weight	Exercise/ Activity	Time	Notes

Exercise Log

Date	Weight	Exercise/ Activity	Time	Notes

Exercise Log

Date	Weight	Exercise/ Activity	Time	Notes

Exercise Log

Date	Weight	Exercise/ Activity	Time	Notes

Exercise Log

Date	Weight	Exercise/ Activity	Time	Notes

Exercise Log

Date	Weight	Exercise/ Activity	Time	Notes

Exercise Log

Date	Weight	Exercise/ Activity	Time	Notes

Exercise Log

Date	Weight	Exercise/ Activity	Time	Notes

Exercise Log

Date	Weight	Exercise/ Activity	Time	Notes

Exercise Log

Date	Weight	Exercise/ Activity	Time	Notes

Exercise Log

Date	Weight	Exercise/ Activity	Time	Notes

Exercise Log

Date	Weight	Exercise/ Activity	Time	Notes

Exercise Log

Date	Weight	Exercise/ Activity	Time	Notes

Exercise Log

Date	Weight	Exercise/ Activity	Time	Notes

Exercise Log

Date	Weight	Exercise/ Activity	Time	Notes

Exercise Log

Date	Weight	Exercise/ Activity	Time	Notes

Exercise Log

Date	Weight	Exercise/ Activity	Time	Notes

Exercise Log

Date	Weight	Exercise/ Activity	Time	Notes

Exercise Log

Date	Weight	Exercise/ Activity	Time	Notes

Exercise Log

Date	Weight	Exercise/ Activity	Time	Notes

Exercise Log

Date	Weight	Exercise/ Activity	Time	Notes

Exercise Log

Date	Weight	Exercise/ Activity	Time	Notes

Exercise Log

Date	Weight	Exercise/ Activity	Time	Notes

Exercise Log

Date	Weight	Exercise/ Activity	Time	Notes

Exercise Log

Date	Weight	Exercise/ Activity	Time	Notes

Exercise Log

Date	Weight	Exercise/ Activity	Time	Notes

Exercise Log

Date	Weight	Exercise/ Activity	Time	Notes

Exercise Log

Date	Weight	Exercise/ Activity	Time	Notes

Exercise Log

Date	Weight	Exercise/ Activity	Time	Notes

Exercise Log

Date	Weight	Exercise/ Activity	Time	Notes

Exercise Log

Date	Weight	Exercise/ Activity	Time	Notes

Exercise Log

Date	Weight	Exercise/ Activity	Time	Notes

Exercise Log

Date	Weight	Exercise/ Activity	Time	Notes

Exercise Log

Date	Weight	Exercise/ Activity	Time	Notes

Exercise Log

Date	Weight	Exercise/ Activity	Time	Notes

Exercise Log

Date	Weight	Exercise/ Activity	Time	Notes

Exercise Log

Date	Weight	Exercise/ Activity	Time	Notes

Exercise Log

Date	Weight	Exercise/ Activity	Time	Notes

Exercise Log

Date	Weight	Exercise/ Activity	Time	Notes

Exercise Log

Date	Weight	Exercise/ Activity	Time	Notes

Exercise Log

Date	Weight	Exercise/ Activity	Time	Notes

Exercise Log

Date	Weight	Exercise/ Activity	Time	Notes

Exercise Log

Date	Weight	Exercise/ Activity	Time	Notes

Exercise Log

Date	Weight	Exercise/ Activity	Time	Notes

Exercise Log

Date	Weight	Exercise/ Activity	Time	Notes

Exercise Log

Date	Weight	Exercise/ Activity	Time	Notes

Exercise Log

Date	Weight	Exercise/ Activity	Time	Notes

Exercise Log

Date	Weight	Exercise/ Activity	Time	Notes

Exercise Log

Date	Weight	Exercise/ Activity	Time	Notes

Exercise Log

Date	Weight	Exercise/ Activity	Time	Notes

Exercise Log

Date	Weight	Exercise/ Activity	Time	Notes

Exercise Log

Date	Weight	Exercise/ Activity	Time	Notes

Exercise Log

Date	Weight	Exercise/ Activity	Time	Notes

Exercise Log

Date	Weight	Exercise/ Activity	Time	Notes

Exercise Log

Date	Weight	Exercise/ Activity	Time	Notes

Exercise Log

Date	Weight	Exercise/ Activity	Time	Notes

Exercise Log

Date	Weight	Exercise/ Activity	Time	Notes

Exercise Log

Date	Weight	Exercise/ Activity	Time	Notes

Exercise Log

Date	Weight	Exercise/ Activity	Time	Notes

Exercise Log

Date	Weight	Exercise/ Activity	Time	Notes

Exercise Log

Date	Weight	Exercise/ Activity	Time	Notes

Exercise Log

Date	Weight	Exercise/ Activity	Time	Notes

Exercise Log

Date	Weight	Exercise/ Activity	Time	Notes

Exercise Log

Date	Weight	Exercise/ Activity	Time	Notes

Exercise Log

Date	Weight	Exercise/ Activity	Time	Notes

Exercise Log

Date	Weight	Exercise/ Activity	Time	Notes

Exercise Log

Date	Weight	Exercise/ Activity	Time	Notes

Exercise Log

Date	Weight	Exercise/ Activity	Time	Notes

Exercise Log

Date	Weight	Exercise/ Activity	Time	Notes

Exercise Log

Date	Weight	Exercise/ Activity	Time	Notes

Exercise Log

Date	Weight	Exercise/ Activity	Time	Notes

Exercise Log

Date	Weight	Exercise/ Activity	Time	Notes

Exercise Log

Date	Weight	Exercise/ Activity	Time	Notes

Exercise Log

Date	Weight	Exercise/ Activity	Time	Notes

Exercise Log

Date	Weight	Exercise/ Activity	Time	Notes

Exercise Log

Date	Weight	Exercise/ Activity	Time	Notes

Exercise Log

Date	Weight	Exercise/ Activity	Time	Notes

Exercise Log

Date	Weight	Exercise/ Activity	Time	Notes

Exercise Log

Date	Weight	Exercise/ Activity	Time	Notes

Exercise Log

Date	Weight	Exercise/Activity	Time	Notes

Exercise Log

Date	Weight	Exercise/ Activity	Time	Notes

Exercise Log

Date	Weight	Exercise/ Activity	Time	Notes

Exercise Log

Date	Weight	Exercise/ Activity	Time	Notes

Exercise Log

Date	Weight	Exercise/ Activity	Time	Notes